Chapter 1: Defining NIK Deficiency

Detailed Definition of NIK Deficiency

NIK deficiency, or NIK (NF-kappa B-inducing kinase) deficiency, is a rare genetic condition that leads to a primary combined T and B cell immunodeficiency. This disorder significantly compromises the immune system, making affected individuals highly susceptible to recurrent and severe viral and bacterial infections. The deficiency arises from mutations in the NIK gene, which plays a crucial role in activating immune responses by regulating the NF-kappa B signaling pathway. This pathway is vital for the development and function of immune cells, particularly T and B lymphocytes, which are essential for adaptive immunity.

Individuals with NIK deficiency typically present with a range of symptoms that can include frequent infections, severe respiratory illnesses, and unusual autoimmune manifestations. The severity and frequency of infections can vary widely among individuals, making early recognition and management critical.

Genetic Basis and Inheritance Patterns

NIK deficiency is inherited in an autosomal recessive manner, which means that an individual must inherit two copies of the mutated gene—one from each parent—to manifest the condition. Parents of an affected individual are usually asymptomatic carriers, possessing one normal and one mutated copy of the NIK gene. Genetic testing can identify carriers and confirm a diagnosis in affected individuals.

Research has indicated that specific mutations in the NIK gene lead to different levels of impairment in immune function. Understanding the genetic basis of NIK deficiency helps researchers explore targeted therapies and potential gene-editing approaches that may one day correct the underlying defect.

Prevalence and Demographics

NIK deficiency is extremely rare, with only a limited number of cases reported in medical literature. Its exact prevalence is difficult to determine due to the rarity of the condition and the fact that many cases may go undiagnosed or misdiagnosed. However, it is believed to affect both males and females equally across diverse ethnic backgrounds.

As awareness of immunodeficiencies has increased, healthcare professionals are becoming more adept at recognizing conditions like NIK deficiency, leading to improved diagnosis rates. Early identification is crucial, as timely intervention can significantly enhance the quality of life for affected individuals and reduce the frequency of infections and related complications.

Importance of Awareness and Understanding

Raising awareness about NIK deficiency is vital for several reasons. First, increased understanding can lead to earlier diagnoses and more effective management strategies. Many individuals with this condition face challenges that can be exacerbated by misinformation or a lack of knowledge among healthcare providers, patients, and families.

Moreover, fostering a supportive community can empower patients and their families to advocate for their health needs, participate in research initiatives, and access appropriate resources. By demystifying NIK deficiency, we can enhance public understanding and promote research efforts that could lead to new treatments.

Goals of the Book

This book aims to provide a comprehensive understanding of NIK deficiency, from its genetic underpinnings to its impact on daily life. By breaking down complex medical information into accessible language, we hope to empower patients, caregivers, and healthcare providers with the knowledge they need to navigate this challenging condition.

Key Goals of This Book:

1. **Educate** readers about the nature and implications of NIK deficiency.
2. **Highlight** the importance of early diagnosis and intervention.
3. **Provide** practical management strategies for daily living.
4. **Foster** a sense of community and support among individuals affected by NIK deficiency.
5. **Encourage** further research and advocacy to improve outcomes for those living with this condition.

Through understanding and mastery of NIK deficiency, we aim to equip affected individuals and their support networks with the tools they need to lead fulfilling lives despite the challenges posed by this rare immunodeficiency.

As we move forward in this book, each subsequent chapter will delve deeper into the complexities of the immune system, the specific challenges associated with NIK deficiency, and the strategies available for managing this condition effectively.

Chapter 2: The Immune System Explained

Overview of the Immune System Components

The immune system is the body's defense network, comprising a complex array of cells, tissues, and organs that work in concert to protect against infections, diseases, and foreign invaders. It can be broadly divided into two main categories: the innate immune system and the adaptive immune system.

Innate Immune System

- **Physical barriers**: Skin and mucous membranes prevent pathogen entry.
- **Phagocytes**: Cells such as macrophages and neutrophils engulf and digest pathogens.
- **Natural killer (NK) cells**: A type of lymphocyte that targets and destroys infected or cancerous cells.
- **Cytokines**: Signaling molecules that mediate and regulate immunity, inflammation, and hematopoiesis.

Adaptive Immune System

T cells

- **Helper T cells (CD4+ T cells)**: Activate and regulate other immune cells.
- **Cytotoxic T cells (CD8+ T cells)**: Directly kill infected or cancerous cells.

B cells

The coordinated efforts of these components ensure that the body can respond effectively to infections and maintain homeostasis.

Role of T and B Cells in Immunity

T and B cells are central players in the adaptive immune response. Their distinct roles are crucial for mounting a robust and effective defense against pathogens.

T Cells

Upon activation by antigen-presenting cells (APCs), T cells undergo clonal expansion and differentiation. Helper T cells enhance the activity of other immune cells, including B cells and cytotoxic T cells, promoting a comprehensive immune response. Cytotoxic T cells directly target and kill infected cells, thereby eliminating the source of infection.

B Cells

B cells are responsible for humoral immunity. When activated by helper T cells or directly by antigens, B cells differentiate into plasma cells that produce antibodies. These antibodies bind to specific antigens on pathogens, neutralizing them and marking them for destruction by other immune cells.

Together, T and B cells provide a highly adaptive and specific immune response, enabling the body to remember past infections and respond more effectively to future encounters with the same pathogens.

How NIK Deficiency Disrupts Normal Immune Function

NIK deficiency disrupts the normal function of both T and B cells due to the crucial role of NIK in the NF-kappa B signaling pathway. This pathway is vital for the activation and survival of various immune cells.

1. **Impaired T Cell Development**: The NIK protein is essential for the proper development and maturation of T cells in the thymus. In NIK deficiency, the signaling required for T cell maturation is compromised, leading to a reduced number of functional T cells. This results in an impaired ability to respond to viral and bacterial infections.

2. **B Cell Dysfunction**: NIK is also important for B cell activation and differentiation. Without functional NIK, B cells may not produce adequate antibodies, resulting in poor humoral responses to infections. This can lead to recurrent bacterial infections and increased susceptibility to diseases that require antibody-mediated immunity.

3. **Increased Susceptibility to Infections**: The combination of reduced T and B cell function means that individuals with NIK deficiency are highly vulnerable to a range of infections, particularly viral and certain bacterial pathogens. The chronic nature of these infections can lead to significant morbidity and may require frequent medical interventions.

4. **Autoimmunity and Inflammation**: Interestingly, some individuals with NIK deficiency may experience autoimmune manifestations due to dysregulated immune responses. The imbalance in immune signaling can lead to inappropriate activation of immune cells, causing them to attack the body's own tissues.

In summary, NIK deficiency severely disrupts normal immune function by impairing the development and activity of T and B cells. This results in increased vulnerability to infections and potential autoimmune complications, underscoring the critical need for awareness, early diagnosis, and effective management strategies.

As we progress through this book, we will explore the specific causes of NIK deficiency, its symptoms, and the various approaches to treatment and management that can help affected individuals lead healthier lives.

Chapter 3: Causes of NIK Deficiency

Genetic Mutations Associated with NIK Deficiency

NIK deficiency is primarily caused by genetic mutations that affect the NIK gene, which encodes for NF-kappa B-inducing kinase (NIK). This protein plays a crucial role in the signaling pathways necessary for the proper function of the immune system. Specifically, NIK is integral to the activation of the NF-kappa B pathway, which regulates the development, survival, and function of immune cells, particularly T and B lymphocytes.

Mutations in the NIK gene can disrupt the normal production or function of the NIK protein, leading to a cascade of immune deficiencies. Various types of mutations can occur, including:

1. **Point Mutations**: These are changes in a single nucleotide base in the DNA sequence of the NIK gene. Point mutations can lead to a nonfunctional or improperly functioning NIK protein.

2. **Insertions and Deletions**: These mutations involve the addition or loss of one or more nucleotides in the NIK gene, which can lead to frameshift mutations. This results in a completely altered protein that is usually nonfunctional.

3. **Copy Number Variations**: In some cases, individuals may have duplications or deletions of the entire NIK gene, leading to either excess or insufficient amounts of NIK protein.

Genetic testing can identify these mutations, confirming a diagnosis of NIK deficiency and providing essential information for family planning and management strategies.

Pathophysiology of the Condition

The pathophysiology of NIK deficiency revolves around the impaired NF-kappa B signaling pathway due to dysfunctional NIK. This disruption leads to several critical consequences:

1. **Impaired Immune Cell Development**: The NIK protein is crucial for the development and maturation of T and B cells. Without functional NIK, the differentiation of these cells is hindered, resulting in a reduced population of mature, functional lymphocytes. This deficiency manifests as a weakened immune response to pathogens.

2. **Inadequate Immune Responses**: With fewer T and B cells, the body struggles to mount effective immune responses. Individuals with NIK deficiency often experience recurrent infections, as their immune systems cannot adequately recognize and combat viruses and bacteria.

3. **Increased Susceptibility to Autoimmunity**: In some cases, the dysregulation of immune signaling due to NIK deficiency can lead to autoimmune issues. The lack of proper immune regulation may cause immune cells to mistakenly attack the body's own tissues, resulting in autoimmune diseases.

4. **Chronic Inflammation**: The altered immune signaling pathways can also contribute to chronic inflammation, further complicating the clinical picture. This inflammation can lead to tissue damage and contribute to the overall burden of disease.

Understanding the underlying pathophysiology of NIK deficiency is crucial for developing targeted therapies and management strategies.

Risk Factors and Environmental Influences

While NIK deficiency is primarily a genetic condition, certain environmental factors and circumstances may influence the severity of symptoms and the frequency of infections:

1. **Infections**: Frequent viral or bacterial infections can exacerbate the symptoms of NIK deficiency. These infections can lead to a cycle of illness, further stressing an already compromised immune system.

2. **Stress**: Psychological and physical stress can impact immune function. Individuals with NIK deficiency may find that stressful situations exacerbate their symptoms or increase their susceptibility to infections.

3. **Nutrition**: Poor nutritional status can further impair immune function. A diet lacking in essential vitamins and minerals may hinder the body's ability to fight infections, particularly in individuals with an already weakened immune system.

4. **Environmental Factors**: Exposure to pollutants, allergens, or other environmental toxins may also play a role in the overall health of individuals with NIK deficiency. These factors can contribute to inflammation and may trigger autoimmune responses in susceptible individuals.

5. **Family History**: Given the genetic nature of NIK deficiency, a family history of immune disorders can also be a risk factor. Individuals with relatives who have similar conditions may be at increased risk of developing NIK deficiency themselves.

In conclusion, NIK deficiency is a complex genetic disorder with significant implications for the immune system. Understanding the genetic mutations and the underlying pathophysiology provides insight into the challenges faced by individuals living with this condition. By recognizing the risk factors and environmental influences that can affect health, we can develop more effective management strategies and improve the quality of life for those affected.

As we delve deeper into the clinical aspects of NIK deficiency in the following chapters, we will explore symptoms, diagnostic procedures, and the importance of early intervention, which are critical for optimizing health outcomes.

Chapter 4: Symptoms and Diagnosis

Common Symptoms

Individuals with NIK deficiency typically experience a range of symptoms, primarily due to their compromised immune system. Recognizing these symptoms early is critical for timely diagnosis and intervention. The most common symptoms include:

Recurrent Infections

- **Viral Infections**: Common colds, influenza, and other viral illnesses may occur more frequently and may last longer.
- **Bacterial Infections**: Patients are particularly susceptible to bacterial infections such as pneumonia, sinusitis, and urinary tract infections. These infections can be severe and may require hospitalization.

2. **Chronic Fatigue**: Persistent fatigue is a common complaint among individuals with NIK deficiency. The body's ongoing battle with infections and the energy expended in immune responses can lead to significant fatigue, impacting daily activities and overall quality of life.

3. **Failure to Thrive**: In children, NIK deficiency may manifest as poor growth or developmental delays. These children may have difficulty gaining weight or meeting developmental milestones due to recurrent illnesses and nutrient malabsorption.

4. **Skin Issues**: Skin rashes and infections may also be prevalent. These can result from the body's inability to fend off pathogens, leading to conditions such as eczema or recurrent skin infections.

5. **Autoimmune Symptoms**: Some individuals may experience symptoms related to autoimmune issues, such as joint pain, swelling, and fatigue. These symptoms arise from the immune system's dysregulation, which can sometimes lead to inappropriate attacks on the body's own tissues.

Diagnostic Procedures

Diagnosing NIK deficiency involves a combination of clinical evaluation, laboratory tests, and genetic analysis. The process typically includes:

1. **Clinical History and Physical Examination**: A thorough medical history, including details about recurrent infections, family history of immune disorders, and any autoimmune symptoms, is critical. A physical examination may reveal signs of infections, growth delays, or skin issues.

2. **Blood Tests**: These tests assess various components of the immune system, including:

- **Complete Blood Count (CBC)**: This test evaluates the overall health of blood cells, including white blood cells (WBCs) that are vital for immune responses.

- **Immunoglobulin Levels**: Measuring levels of different types of immunoglobulins (antibodies) can help determine if the body is producing adequate immune responses.

3. **Genetic Testing**: If NIK deficiency is suspected, genetic testing is essential to confirm the diagnosis. This may involve sequencing the NIK gene to identify specific mutations. Genetic counseling may also be recommended to discuss the implications of the findings for the patient and their family.

4. **Functional Assays**: In some cases, functional tests may be conducted to assess the immune system's capability to respond to stimuli. This can include testing how well T and B cells proliferate and produce antibodies in response to antigens.

Importance of Early Diagnosis

Early diagnosis of NIK deficiency is crucial for several reasons:

1. **Timely Interventions**: Identifying NIK deficiency early allows for prompt implementation of treatments, such as immunoglobulin replacement therapy and prophylactic antibiotics. These measures can help prevent severe infections and improve the quality of life.

2. **Preventing Complications**: Early detection can minimize the risk of complications associated with recurrent infections, such as lung damage or chronic sinusitis. It also helps in managing any potential autoimmune symptoms before they escalate.

3. **Family Planning and Genetic Counseling**: For families with a known history of NIK deficiency, early diagnosis can guide reproductive choices and provide valuable information about the risk of passing on the condition to future children.

4. **Support and Resources**: Early diagnosis connects individuals and families with support resources, including healthcare providers specializing in immunodeficiencies, support groups, and educational materials. This support is vital for navigating the challenges associated with living with NIK deficiency.

In conclusion, recognizing the symptoms of NIK deficiency and understanding the diagnostic process are critical steps toward effective management of the condition. As we move forward in this book, we will delve into the complications that can arise from NIK deficiency and explore treatment options that can significantly improve outcomes for affected individuals.

Chapter 5: Complications of NIK Deficiency

Short-Term Complications

Individuals with NIK deficiency face a variety of short-term complications primarily stemming from their increased susceptibility to infections. These complications can significantly impact their health and daily functioning. Key short-term complications include:

1. **Severe Infections**: Recurrent viral and bacterial infections can be particularly severe. Patients may experience pneumonia, recurrent ear infections, and frequent respiratory infections that require hospitalization. These infections can lead to complications like sepsis or chronic lung disease, especially in young children.

2. **Delayed Recovery**: The immune system's impaired response often results in prolonged illness. Recovery from infections may take significantly longer compared to individuals with a fully functioning immune system. This can lead to additional health challenges and increased healthcare costs.

3. **Hospitalization**: Due to the severity of infections and the risk of complications, many individuals with NIK deficiency may require frequent hospital visits or extended stays. Hospitalization can pose its own risks, including exposure to nosocomial infections and the psychological impact of being hospitalized frequently.

4. **Invasive Procedures**: In some cases, recurrent infections may necessitate invasive procedures such as intravenous (IV) antibiotic administration, which can be uncomfortable and carry risks of complications like phlebitis or catheter-related infections.

Long-Term Complications

Long-term complications of NIK deficiency can have profound effects on an individual's health and quality of life. These may include:

1. **Chronic Health Issues**: Individuals may develop chronic conditions as a result of frequent infections or prolonged immune dysregulation. Chronic lung disease, for example, can result from repeated respiratory infections, leading to lasting pulmonary complications.

2. **Autoimmune Disorders**: The immune dysregulation associated with NIK deficiency can lead to the development of autoimmune diseases. Patients may experience conditions such as rheumatoid arthritis or lupus, resulting in additional health challenges and requiring further medical management.

3. **Growth and Developmental Delays**: In children, chronic infections and the energy expended fighting these illnesses can lead to growth delays and developmental challenges. These may affect physical, cognitive, and emotional development, necessitating additional support services.

4. **Psychosocial Implications**: Living with a chronic condition like NIK deficiency can lead to social isolation, anxiety, and depression. The stress of managing a complex health condition can affect mental health, leading to long-term emotional challenges.

Impact on Quality of Life

The complications associated with NIK deficiency profoundly impact quality of life. Factors influencing this impact include:

1. **Physical Limitations**: Frequent infections and their complications can limit physical activity, resulting in decreased stamina and fitness. Individuals may struggle to keep up with peers in school or social settings, leading to feelings of frustration and isolation.

2. **Educational Challenges**: Children with NIK deficiency may miss significant amounts of school due to illness, affecting their academic performance and social interactions. This can result in educational delays, requiring additional educational support and resources.

3. **Financial Burden**: The cost of ongoing medical care, frequent hospital visits, and medications can create a significant financial burden for families. This economic stress can compound the emotional and physical challenges associated with the condition.

4. **Family Dynamics**: The impact of NIK deficiency extends beyond the individual. Family members often experience stress related to caregiving, navigating healthcare systems, and managing the emotional toll of living with a chronic illness. Family support and resources can be critical in mitigating these challenges.

Coexisting Conditions

Individuals with NIK deficiency may also experience coexisting conditions that complicate their clinical management. Some common coexisting issues include:

1. **Allergic Conditions**: Many individuals with NIK deficiency have a higher prevalence of allergies, including asthma and eczema. These conditions can complicate management and further strain the immune system.

2. **Gastrointestinal Issues**: Chronic gastrointestinal symptoms, such as diarrhea or malabsorption, may occur due to recurrent infections or dysbiosis in gut microbiota. This can lead to nutritional deficiencies and further exacerbate immune dysfunction.

3. **Mental Health Disorders**: Anxiety and depression are common among individuals with chronic illnesses, including NIK deficiency. The psychological burden of frequent illness and the stress of managing a complex health condition can lead to long-term mental health challenges.

Conclusion

The complications of NIK deficiency, both short-term and long-term, underscore the importance of comprehensive management strategies. Understanding these complications can help healthcare providers and families anticipate potential challenges and take proactive steps to address them. As we continue through this book, we will explore treatment options that can mitigate these complications and enhance the quality of life for those affected by NIK deficiency. By equipping individuals and families with knowledge and resources, we can foster resilience and empower them in their journey toward mastering NIK deficiency.

Chapter 6: Treatment Options

Overview of Current Treatments

Managing NIK deficiency requires a comprehensive approach tailored to each individual's unique needs. Current treatment options aim to reduce the frequency and severity of infections, bolster immune function, and improve overall quality of life. This chapter discusses the primary treatment modalities, their mechanisms of action, and considerations for patients and caregivers.

Immunoglobulin Replacement Therapy

One of the cornerstone treatments for individuals with NIK deficiency is **immunoglobulin replacement therapy (IRT)**. This therapy involves the administration of immunoglobulins, which are antibodies derived from the plasma of healthy donors.

Mechanism of Action

1. **Restoration of Antibody Levels**: IRT helps to restore immunoglobulin levels in patients, providing them with the necessary antibodies to fight infections.

2. **Passive Immunity**: The antibodies from donor plasma can offer immediate passive immunity against specific pathogens that the patient may not be able to effectively combat due to their deficiency.

Administration

Immunoglobulin therapy can be administered through two primary methods:

- **Intravenous (IV) Administration**: This method involves infusing immunoglobulins directly into the bloodstream, usually in a clinical setting.

- **Subcutaneous (SC) Administration**: Patients can also self-administer immunoglobulins under the skin, which may be more convenient for some and allow for more frequent dosing.

Frequency and Dosing

The frequency of IRT can vary based on individual needs but typically ranges from every few weeks to monthly. Dosing is individualized based on the patient's weight, age, and immunoglobulin levels.

Benefits and Considerations

- **Benefits**: Patients often experience fewer infections and reduced severity when infections do occur.

- **Considerations**: Potential side effects include allergic reactions, headaches, and, in rare cases, kidney complications. Close monitoring is essential to mitigate these risks.

Use of Antibiotics and Antivirals

Given the recurrent infections associated with NIK deficiency, the proactive use of antibiotics and antiviral medications plays a vital role in treatment.

Antibiotic Prophylaxis

1. **Prophylactic Antibiotics**: For patients with frequent bacterial infections, healthcare providers may prescribe prophylactic antibiotics. These medications help prevent infections before they occur.

2. **Targeted Therapy**: When infections do arise, targeted antibiotic therapy based on the specific bacteria causing the infection is critical for effective treatment.

Antiviral Treatments

1. **Preventive Antivirals**: In cases where patients are prone to viral infections, preventive antiviral medications may be prescribed, especially during outbreaks of specific viruses (e.g., influenza).

2. **Treatment During Infections**: If a viral infection occurs, antiviral medications can help manage the symptoms and reduce the duration of the illness.

Supportive Care

In addition to immunoglobulin therapy and antimicrobial agents, supportive care measures are essential for overall health management.

Nutritional Support

- **Balanced Diet**: A well-rounded diet rich in vitamins and minerals supports immune function. Nutritional consultations can provide personalized dietary recommendations.
- **Supplements**: In some cases, nutritional supplements, such as vitamin D or zinc, may be recommended to bolster immune health.

Symptomatic Management

- **Management of Symptoms**: Addressing symptoms of infections, such as fever and pain, with appropriate medications can enhance comfort and quality of life.
- **Physical Therapy**: For patients with chronic lung issues or fatigue, physical therapy can improve strength and endurance, facilitating better overall health.

Emerging Therapies and Research

Research is ongoing to explore new treatment modalities for NIK deficiency. Potential advancements include:

1. **Gene Therapy**: Innovative gene therapies aim to correct the underlying genetic mutations responsible for NIK deficiency, offering hope for long-term solutions.

2. **Monoclonal Antibodies**: These laboratory-engineered antibodies target specific pathogens more effectively than traditional immunoglobulin therapy, potentially providing enhanced protection.

3. **Personalized Medicine**: As our understanding of the immune system evolves, treatment approaches may increasingly become personalized based on genetic and immunological profiles.

Conclusion

Effective management of NIK deficiency hinges on a multifaceted treatment strategy. Immunoglobulin replacement therapy, antibiotics, and supportive care form the backbone of care, while ongoing research holds promise for future advancements. By working closely with healthcare providers, individuals with NIK deficiency can create tailored treatment plans that address their unique challenges, ultimately enhancing their quality of life and resilience against infections. As we progress through this book, we will explore management strategies and lifestyle adjustments that further empower individuals in their journey to master NIK deficiency.

Chapter 7: Management Strategies

Effective management of NIK deficiency is multifaceted, involving a blend of personalized care plans, interdisciplinary collaboration, and ongoing monitoring. This chapter outlines key strategies to ensure that individuals with NIK deficiency can lead healthier lives, minimize complications, and maximize their overall well-being.

Individualized Care Plans
Personalization of Treatment

Each person with NIK deficiency presents a unique profile of symptoms, health status, and needs. Therefore, an **individualized care plan** is essential.

Assessment of Needs

- Medical history
- Frequency and types of infections
- Response to previous treatments
- Psychosocial factors affecting health

Goal Setting

- Reducing the frequency of infections
- Enhancing physical activity levels
- Improving mental health

Intervention Planning

- Adjustments to immunoglobulin therapy

- Prophylactic antibiotics

- Nutritional support tailored to individual dietary needs

Flexibility in Care

Individualized plans should remain flexible to adapt to changing circumstances, such as:

- New health challenges

- Changes in lifestyle or environment

- Advances in treatment options

Importance of Multidisciplinary Teams

A **multidisciplinary approach** brings together diverse expertise to address the various aspects of managing NIK deficiency. Key team members may include:

1. **Immunologists**: Specialists who understand the intricacies of immune disorders and can tailor immunotherapy.

2. **Infectious Disease Specialists**: Experts in managing and preventing infections that individuals with NIK deficiency may face.

3. **Nutritionists/Dietitians**: Professionals who can design nutrition plans to bolster immune health and overall well-being.

4. **Psychologists/Psychiatrists**: Mental health professionals to support emotional resilience and coping strategies for the psychological impacts of living with a chronic condition.

5. **Primary Care Providers**: Coordinators of care who ensure that all team members communicate effectively and that patients receive comprehensive support.

Communication and Collaboration

Regular meetings and communication among team members facilitate coordinated care. This collaborative environment helps ensure that all aspects of the patient's health are considered, promoting a holistic approach to treatment.

Regular Monitoring and Follow-Up

Ongoing monitoring is crucial for optimizing care and improving health outcomes.

Routine Assessments

1. **Health Check-ups**: Regular visits to healthcare providers help track health changes, assess treatment efficacy, and adjust care plans as needed.

2. **Laboratory Tests**: Routine blood tests can monitor immunoglobulin levels, identify infections early, and assess organ function.

3. **Vaccination Updates**: Staying current with vaccinations is critical for preventing infections, especially for individuals with weakened immune systems.

Emergency Planning

Emergency Protocols

- Instructions on when to seek immediate care
- Emergency contact information for healthcare providers
- Medication lists and allergy information

Education on Warning Signs

Empowering Patients and Caregivers

Encouraging patient and caregiver involvement in management strategies fosters empowerment and enhances treatment adherence.

1. **Education**: Provide resources and training on NIK deficiency, treatment options, and self-care strategies. Understanding the condition empowers individuals to take an active role in their health.

2. **Support Networks**: Encourage participation in support groups or communities for individuals with NIK deficiency. Sharing experiences and coping strategies can provide emotional support and practical advice.

3. **Self-Management Skills**: Teach self-management techniques, including:

- Monitoring symptoms
- Recognizing when to seek medical help
- Implementing lifestyle adjustments to support health

Conclusion

Effective management of NIK deficiency relies on a comprehensive, individualized approach that includes tailored care plans, multidisciplinary collaboration, and regular monitoring. By engaging patients and their families in the management process and leveraging a supportive healthcare network, individuals with NIK deficiency can improve their quality of life and health outcomes. As we continue through this book, we will explore additional lifestyle adjustments and psychological strategies to further support those living with this condition.

Chapter 8: Lifestyle Adjustments

Managing NIK deficiency effectively involves not only medical treatments but also lifestyle adjustments that can significantly enhance overall health and well-being. This chapter explores key areas where individuals and families can make proactive changes to support immune health and reduce the risk of complications associated with NIK deficiency.

Nutrition and Immune Health

A well-balanced diet plays a critical role in supporting the immune system, especially for individuals with NIK deficiency. Here are important nutritional considerations:

Balanced Diet

1. **Nutrient-Rich Foods**: Focus on incorporating a variety of fruits, vegetables, whole grains, lean proteins, and healthy fats into daily meals. These foods provide essential vitamins and minerals that are vital for immune function.

2. **Key Nutrients**:

- **Vitamin C**: Found in citrus fruits, strawberries, and bell peppers, vitamin C is crucial for the growth and repair of tissues and helps combat oxidative stress.

- **Vitamin D**: Important for immune health, vitamin D can be sourced from fatty fish, fortified dairy products, and exposure to sunlight. Supplementation may be necessary for individuals with low levels.

- **Zinc**: Present in meats, shellfish, legumes, and seeds, zinc supports the development and function of immune cells.

Hydration

Staying hydrated is essential for overall health. Water helps in transporting nutrients and maintaining bodily functions. Aim for adequate fluid intake throughout the day, adjusting for activity levels and environmental conditions.

Dietary Supplements

In some cases, dietary supplements may be recommended to fill nutritional gaps. Always consult with a healthcare provider before starting any supplementation to ensure safety and efficacy.

Importance of Hygiene and Infection Control

Individuals with NIK deficiency are at an increased risk for infections. Implementing stringent hygiene practices can help reduce this risk significantly.

Hand Hygiene

1. **Frequent Handwashing**: Regularly washing hands with soap and water, especially before meals and after using the restroom, can help prevent the spread of germs.
2. **Use of Hand Sanitizers**: When soap and water are not available, alcohol-based hand sanitizers can be effective in reducing germs on hands.

Environmental Cleanliness

1. **Regular Cleaning**: Keep living spaces clean by regularly disinfecting surfaces, especially those frequently touched (doorknobs, countertops, and electronics).

2. **Avoiding Crowded Places**: Limit exposure to crowded environments during peak infection seasons to reduce the risk of contracting illnesses.

Vaccination

Staying up to date with vaccinations is crucial for individuals with weakened immune systems. Discuss appropriate vaccines with a healthcare provider, including annual flu shots and other recommended immunizations.

Physical Activity Considerations

Maintaining an active lifestyle is important for both physical and mental health. Regular exercise can boost the immune system, improve energy levels, and enhance overall quality of life.

Exercise Recommendations

1. **Moderate Activity**: Aim for at least 150 minutes of moderate aerobic activity per week, such as walking, swimming, or cycling. This can help improve cardiovascular health and boost immunity.

2. **Strength Training**: Include muscle-strengthening activities at least two days per week. This can enhance physical strength, improve metabolism, and support bone health.

3. **Flexibility and Balance**: Incorporate stretching and balance exercises, such as yoga or tai chi, to improve flexibility and reduce the risk of injury.

Listening to Your Body

It's essential to tailor physical activity to individual capabilities. If fatigue or other symptoms arise, it's important to adjust the level of activity and consult with healthcare providers as needed.

Stress Management

Chronic stress can negatively impact the immune system. Implementing stress management techniques can be beneficial.

Mindfulness and Relaxation Techniques

1. **Mindfulness Meditation**: Practicing mindfulness can help reduce stress and improve emotional well-being. Consider guided meditation apps or local classes.
2. **Deep Breathing Exercises**: Simple breathing exercises can be performed anywhere and help alleviate stress quickly.
3. **Engaging in Hobbies**: Pursuing enjoyable activities and hobbies can provide a sense of purpose and relaxation.

Conclusion

Lifestyle adjustments are a vital part of managing NIK deficiency and supporting immune health. By focusing on nutrition, hygiene, physical activity, and stress management, individuals can significantly enhance their overall quality of life. These strategies, combined with medical treatments, create a holistic approach to living well with NIK deficiency. As we move forward in this book, we will delve into the psychological impact of living with this condition and explore effective coping strategies to promote emotional resilience.

Chapter 9: Psychological Impact

Living with NIK deficiency can take a toll not only on physical health but also on emotional and psychological well-being. Understanding these impacts and exploring effective coping strategies are essential for enhancing quality of life. This chapter delves into the emotional challenges faced by individuals with NIK deficiency and offers insights into resilience and support systems.

Emotional and Psychological Effects
Anxiety and Stress

The uncertainty associated with managing a chronic condition like NIK deficiency can lead to heightened levels of anxiety and stress. Concerns about recurrent infections, treatment efficacy, and the impact on daily life can create a persistent sense of worry.

- **Fear of Illness**: The potential for frequent infections can lead to a constant vigilance about health, which may exacerbate anxiety.
- **Stress from Treatment Regimens**: Adhering to complex treatment plans can be overwhelming, contributing to feelings of frustration and helplessness.

Depression

Individuals with NIK deficiency may experience depression due to the challenges of living with a chronic illness. Symptoms can include:

- **Loss of Interest**: A decrease in interest in activities once enjoyed.
- **Feelings of Isolation**: Chronic illness can lead to social withdrawal, making individuals feel isolated from friends and family.

Impact on Self-Identity

Living with NIK deficiency can alter one's self-perception. The struggle with health may lead to feelings of inadequacy or a sense of being different from peers, which can affect self-esteem.

Strategies for Coping and Resilience

Developing coping mechanisms is crucial for managing the psychological impact of NIK deficiency. Here are several effective strategies:

Emotional Awareness and Expression

1. **Recognizing Emotions**: Encourage awareness of one's feelings and experiences. Keeping a journal can help in identifying patterns of mood and triggers for anxiety or depression.

2. **Expressing Feelings**: Talking about emotions with trusted friends, family, or a therapist can provide relief and clarity. Creative outlets, such as art or music, can also serve as valuable forms of expression.

Building Resilience

1. **Positive Thinking**: Cultivating a positive mindset can significantly affect emotional well-being. Focus on strengths and achievements, no matter how small.

2. **Setting Realistic Goals**: Establishing achievable short-term goals can foster a sense of accomplishment and purpose.

3. **Mindfulness and Relaxation**: Incorporate mindfulness practices such as meditation, deep breathing exercises, or yoga to reduce stress and promote mental clarity.

Seeking Professional Help

Engaging with mental health professionals can provide additional support. Therapy options may include:

- **Cognitive Behavioral Therapy (CBT)**: This approach can help individuals reframe negative thought patterns and develop healthier coping strategies.
- **Support Groups**: Connecting with others who share similar experiences can provide comfort and a sense of community. Sharing stories can reduce feelings of isolation.

Support Systems and Resources

Having a robust support system is vital for emotional health. Here are some ways to enhance support:

Family and Friends

Educating family and friends about NIK deficiency is crucial. Open communication fosters understanding and empathy, enabling loved ones to offer better support.

Support Groups and Community Resources

1. **Local Support Groups**: These groups provide opportunities to meet others facing similar challenges, share experiences, and gain valuable insights. Look for groups specifically for individuals with immune deficiencies or chronic health conditions.

2. **Online Communities**: Social media platforms and dedicated online forums can connect individuals with a wider network of support, offering a space to share experiences and advice.

3. **Mental Health Resources**: Many organizations offer resources specifically aimed at supporting individuals with chronic illnesses. Consider reaching out to local or national health organizations for guidance and support.

Conclusion

Understanding and addressing the psychological impact of NIK deficiency is essential for fostering resilience and promoting overall well-being. By recognizing emotional challenges, developing coping strategies, and utilizing support systems, individuals can navigate the complexities of living with this condition more effectively. In the next chapter, we will explore practical day-to-day management tips for living with NIK deficiency, emphasizing strategies for education and preparedness.

Chapter 10: Living with NIK Deficiency

Living with NIK deficiency requires a proactive approach to manage health effectively while maintaining a fulfilling lifestyle. This chapter focuses on practical day-to-day management tips, the importance of education for family and friends, and strategies for preparing for medical emergencies.

Day-to-Day Management Tips

1. Establishing a Routine

Creating a consistent daily routine can provide stability and help in managing symptoms. Key components include:

- **Medication Management**: Keep a schedule for medications and treatments, using pill organizers or reminders on your phone to ensure adherence.
- **Nutrition**: Plan balanced meals that support immune health. Include a variety of fruits, vegetables, whole grains, and lean proteins in your diet.

2. Monitoring Health

Regular health monitoring is crucial for managing NIK deficiency effectively:

- **Symptom Tracking**: Maintain a health journal to track symptoms, treatments, and any side effects. This information can be invaluable for discussions with healthcare providers.
- **Regular Check-Ups**: Schedule routine appointments with your healthcare team to monitor your condition and adjust treatments as needed.

3. Prioritizing Self-Care

Taking care of your mental and physical well-being is essential:

- **Stress Management**: Incorporate stress-relief practices into your routine, such as mindfulness, meditation, or hobbies that bring joy.
- **Adequate Rest**: Ensure you get sufficient sleep each night to help your body recover and function optimally.

Educating Family and Friends

1. Open Communication

Having open discussions about NIK deficiency with family and friends fosters understanding and support. Consider:

- **Explaining the Condition**: Share information about NIK deficiency, its symptoms, and its impact on daily life. This can help loved ones understand what you are going through.
- **Encouraging Questions**: Invite questions to clarify any misconceptions and promote empathy.

2. Involvement in Care

Engaging family and friends in your care plan can create a supportive environment:

- **Treatment Support**: Inform them about your treatment schedule and how they can help, whether it's reminding you to take medications or accompanying you to appointments.
- **Participating in Activities**: Encourage loved ones to participate in healthy activities with you, such as cooking nutritious meals or exercising together.

Preparing for Medical Emergencies

Being prepared for medical emergencies is vital for anyone with a chronic condition like NIK deficiency. Here are steps to take:

1. Creating a Medical Emergency Kit

Prepare a kit that includes essential items:

- **Medication List**: Keep an updated list of medications, dosages, and any allergies. Include contact information for your healthcare providers.
- **Emergency Contacts**: List emergency contacts, including family members, friends, and healthcare professionals, and keep this information easily accessible.

2. Developing an Action Plan

Having a clear action plan can help during emergencies:

- **Recognizing Symptoms**: Know which symptoms require immediate medical attention, such as signs of severe infection.
- **Emergency Procedures**: Outline what to do in various situations, including how to reach medical help quickly.

3. Educating Others

Make sure that family and friends are aware of the emergency action plan:

- **Role-Playing Scenarios**: Consider conducting mock scenarios to practice what to do in case of an emergency.
- **Sharing Information**: Ensure that key people in your life have access to your medical information and understand how to respond effectively.

Conclusion

Living with NIK deficiency involves a comprehensive approach to daily management, education, and preparation for emergencies. By establishing routines, fostering open communication, and being prepared for medical situations, individuals can lead fulfilling lives while effectively managing their condition. In the next chapter, we will explore advances in research related to immunodeficiencies, highlighting promising developments that may shape future treatment options.

Chapter 11: Advances in Research

Research into NIK deficiency and related immunodeficiencies is continually evolving, offering hope for improved treatments and better understanding of these complex conditions. This chapter explores current research trends, innovative therapies like gene therapy, and the importance of clinical trials in shaping the future of NIK deficiency management.

Current Research Trends in Immunodeficiencies

1. Understanding the Genetic Basis

Recent studies have focused on identifying specific genetic mutations associated with NIK deficiency. Researchers are using advanced genomic technologies, such as whole-exome sequencing, to uncover the underlying genetic mechanisms. This knowledge not only helps in diagnosing NIK deficiency earlier but also provides insights into potential therapeutic targets.

2. Immune System Functionality

Investigations into how NIK deficiency affects immune system functionality are ongoing. Studies are examining the roles of various immune cells, including T and B cells, and how their interactions are altered in individuals with NIK deficiency. Understanding these dynamics is crucial for developing targeted treatments that can restore normal immune function.

3. Biomarkers for Disease Monitoring

Research is also focused on identifying biomarkers that can help monitor the disease's progression and response to treatment. Biomarkers can provide objective measures of immune function, making it easier for healthcare providers to tailor therapies and predict outcomes for patients.

Gene Therapy and Potential Future Treatments
1. The Promise of Gene Therapy

Gene therapy represents a groundbreaking approach for treating genetic conditions, including NIK deficiency. By correcting or replacing the defective gene responsible for the condition, researchers aim to restore normal immune function. Early clinical trials have shown promising results, but more extensive studies are needed to assess safety and efficacy.

Case Studies

2. CRISPR Technology

The advent of CRISPR-Cas9 technology has opened new avenues for gene editing in NIK deficiency research. This powerful tool allows for precise modifications of genetic sequences, potentially correcting mutations that cause immune dysfunction. Researchers are exploring its application in laboratory settings, and initial findings are encouraging.

Importance of Clinical Trials

1. Advancing Treatment Options

Clinical trials are essential for evaluating new therapies and improving existing treatment protocols for NIK deficiency. Participation in clinical trials offers patients access to cutting-edge treatments and contributes to the broader understanding of the condition.

Finding Trials

2. Patient Advocacy in Research

Advocacy plays a crucial role in advancing research. Patients, families, and advocacy organizations can help raise awareness about the importance of research funding and participation in clinical trials. By sharing their experiences and challenges, they can influence research priorities and promote studies that focus on real-world patient needs.

Conclusion

The landscape of research on NIK deficiency is dynamic, with significant advancements being made in understanding its genetic basis, exploring innovative treatments like gene therapy, and emphasizing the importance of clinical trials. As research continues to evolve, the hope for improved management strategies and potential cures becomes increasingly tangible. In the next chapter, we will explore how to navigate healthcare systems effectively, ensuring that individuals with NIK deficiency receive the care and support they need.

Chapter 12: Navigating Healthcare Systems

Navigating the healthcare system can be daunting, especially for those living with NIK deficiency. Understanding healthcare rights, effective communication strategies, and advocacy resources is essential for ensuring that individuals receive the best possible care. This chapter provides guidance on how to successfully maneuver through the complexities of healthcare systems.

Understanding Healthcare Rights and Access

1. Patient Rights

Every patient has rights that protect their access to healthcare, including the right to receive appropriate medical treatment, privacy, and informed consent. Key rights include:

- **Right to Information**: Patients should have access to all relevant medical information and understand their treatment options.
- **Right to Non-Discrimination**: Patients cannot be denied treatment based on their condition, including NIK deficiency.
- **Right to Privacy**: Patients have the right to keep their medical information confidential.

Familiarizing yourself with these rights can empower you and help ensure you receive fair treatment.

2. Accessing Care

Accessing specialized care for NIK deficiency may require navigating multiple healthcare facilities and providers. Here are some tips:

- **Research Specialists**: Identify healthcare providers who specialize in immunodeficiencies or NIK deficiency. Academic medical centers often have experts in these fields.
- **Referral Networks**: Work with your primary care physician to obtain referrals to specialists. Ensure they understand the urgency and specific needs related to NIK deficiency.

Tips for Effective Communication with Healthcare Providers

1. Prepare for Appointments

Preparation is key to effective communication:

- **Gather Medical Records**: Bring all relevant medical records, including previous test results and treatment plans, to appointments.
- **Create a List of Questions**: Write down any questions or concerns you have about your condition or treatment options.

2. Be Clear and Concise

During appointments, communicate clearly:

- **Describe Symptoms Accurately**: Be specific about your symptoms, their frequency, and how they impact your daily life.
- **Express Your Goals**: Let your healthcare provider know your treatment goals and what you hope to achieve from the visit.

3. Advocate for Yourself

Sometimes, you may need to advocate for more comprehensive care:

- **Request Further Tests**: If you feel that additional testing is warranted, discuss this with your provider.
- **Seek a Second Opinion**: If you are unsure about a diagnosis or treatment plan, don't hesitate to seek a second opinion from another specialist.

Advocacy for Improved Care and Awareness

1. Getting Involved

Advocacy can play a vital role in improving care for individuals with NIK deficiency:

- **Join Advocacy Groups**: Organizations focused on immunodeficiencies often have resources, support networks, and opportunities for advocacy.
- **Participate in Awareness Campaigns**: Engaging in campaigns can help raise awareness and improve understanding of NIK deficiency within the healthcare community.

2. Educating Healthcare Providers

Many healthcare providers may not be familiar with NIK deficiency. Consider:

- **Providing Educational Materials**: Bring brochures or articles about NIK deficiency to appointments, especially if your provider is less familiar with the condition.
- **Sharing Your Story**: Personal experiences can help providers understand the challenges faced by patients with NIK deficiency, leading to more empathetic and informed care.

Conclusion

Navigating healthcare systems requires awareness of your rights, effective communication skills, and a proactive approach to advocacy. By understanding the intricacies of healthcare access and building strong relationships with healthcare providers, individuals with NIK deficiency can secure the care and support they need. In the next chapter, we will explore the vital role of support groups in providing community and resources for those affected by NIK deficiency.

Chapter 13: The Role of Support Groups

Support groups play a vital role in the lives of individuals affected by NIK deficiency. These communities provide not only emotional support but also practical resources, education, and a sense of belonging. In this chapter, we will explore the benefits of joining support groups, how to find and participate in these communities, and the importance of sharing experiences and advice.

Benefits of Joining Support Groups

1. Emotional Support

Living with NIK deficiency can be isolating, and connecting with others who share similar experiences can be incredibly validating. Support groups offer:

- **A Safe Space**: Members can share their feelings, concerns, and triumphs without fear of judgment.
- **Shared Understanding**: Fellow members understand the nuances of living with NIK deficiency, providing empathy and encouragement.

2. Practical Resources

Support groups often serve as a hub for sharing valuable information:

- **Access to Information**: Members can exchange tips on managing symptoms, navigating healthcare systems, and finding specialists.
- **Resource Sharing**: Groups may provide materials or recommend books, websites, and other resources focused on NIK deficiency.

3. Advocacy and Awareness

Support groups can also be powerful advocates for change:

- **Collective Voice**: By banding together, members can raise awareness about NIK deficiency and push for better healthcare access and policies.
- **Educational Outreach**: Groups may engage in community education initiatives to inform the public about the condition.

How to Find and Participate in Local and Online Communities

1. Searching for Support Groups

Finding the right support group can make all the difference. Here are some strategies:

- **Online Resources**: Websites like the Immune Deficiency Foundation and local health organizations often list support groups and forums.
- **Social Media**: Platforms like Facebook, Reddit, and specialized forums can connect you with virtual support groups focused on NIK deficiency.
- **Healthcare Providers**: Ask your doctor or specialist for recommendations on local support groups.

2. Engaging in the Community

Once you find a group, participating actively can enhance your experience:

- **Attend Meetings**: Whether in-person or virtual, regular attendance helps build relationships and deepen connections.
- **Share Your Story**: Personal experiences can be incredibly impactful. Sharing your journey can inspire and help others in similar situations.
- **Ask Questions**: Don't hesitate to seek advice or clarification on issues you're facing. Support groups thrive on mutual assistance.

Sharing Experiences and Advice

The collective wisdom within support groups can be a rich resource:

1. Learning from Others

Hearing others' experiences can provide insights into managing NIK deficiency effectively:

- **Coping Strategies**: Members may share techniques that have worked for them in dealing with symptoms or emotional challenges.
- **Success Stories**: Sharing positive experiences can offer hope and motivation to others facing difficulties.

2. Providing Support

You don't just receive support; you also contribute to the community:

- **Offering Advice**: If you've found effective strategies or resources, sharing these can be incredibly helpful to others.
- **Being a Mentor**: As you gain experience, consider mentoring newer members who may be feeling lost or overwhelmed.

Conclusion

Support groups are invaluable for individuals living with NIK deficiency. They offer emotional comfort, practical resources, and a platform for advocacy. By finding and actively participating in these communities, you not only enhance your own experience but also contribute to the collective strength of those affected by NIK deficiency. In the next chapter, we will discuss the importance of education and awareness in improving understanding and support for individuals with this condition.

Chapter 14: Education and Awareness

Education and awareness are critical in addressing the challenges faced by individuals with NIK deficiency. By fostering a greater understanding of this condition, we can improve support, reduce stigma, and promote better health outcomes. This chapter will explore the importance of educating the public, strategies for raising awareness in your community, and the role of social media and campaigns in this endeavor.

Importance of Educating the Public about NIK Deficiency

1. Reducing Stigma

NIK deficiency, like many immunodeficiencies, can be misunderstood. Education plays a vital role in:

- **Challenging Misconceptions**: Many people may not understand what NIK deficiency is or how it affects individuals. By educating others, we can dispel myths and reduce fear associated with the condition.
- **Promoting Empathy**: A better understanding of NIK deficiency fosters compassion and support, making it easier for affected individuals to navigate their daily lives.

2. Encouraging Early Diagnosis

Increased awareness can lead to:

- **Improved Recognition**: Educating healthcare professionals and the general public can help ensure earlier identification of symptoms, leading to timely diagnosis and treatment.
- **Access to Resources**: Greater awareness can result in more resources being allocated for research, healthcare, and support services.

3. Empowering Individuals

Education empowers those affected by NIK deficiency:

- **Knowledge is Power**: Understanding their condition helps individuals make informed decisions about their health and treatment options.
- **Community Building**: Educated individuals are more likely to connect with others facing similar challenges, fostering support networks.

Strategies for Raising Awareness in Your Community

1. Organizing Educational Events

Hosting community events can be an effective way to spread knowledge:

- **Workshops and Seminars**: Collaborate with healthcare providers to hold informational sessions about NIK deficiency, its symptoms, and management strategies.
- **Health Fairs**: Participate in local health fairs to distribute educational materials and engage with the public directly.

2. Partnering with Local Organizations

Collaborating with established organizations can amplify your efforts:

- **Schools and Universities**: Work with educational institutions to incorporate information about NIK deficiency into health education curricula.
- **Nonprofits and Advocacy Groups**: Partner with organizations dedicated to immunodeficiencies to co-host events or create awareness campaigns.

3. Utilizing Media Outlets

Media can be a powerful tool for spreading awareness:

- **Press Releases**: Create press releases for local newspapers or radio stations to highlight awareness events or initiatives.
- **Interviews and Articles**: Seek opportunities to be featured in interviews or write articles about NIK deficiency for community publications.

Role of Social Media and Campaigns

1. Engaging Online Communities

Social media platforms offer a unique space for education and outreach:

- **Creating Dedicated Pages**: Establish dedicated social media pages to share information, resources, and personal stories related to NIK deficiency.
- **Hashtag Campaigns**: Develop and promote specific hashtags to raise awareness and encourage discussions around NIK deficiency.

2. Sharing Personal Stories

Personal narratives can humanize the condition:

- **Storytelling**: Encourage individuals to share their experiences with NIK deficiency online. Personal stories resonate with audiences and foster understanding.
- **Video Campaigns**: Utilize platforms like YouTube or TikTok to create video content that explains NIK deficiency, showcasing real-life experiences and challenges.

3. Collaborating with Influencers

Engaging with social media influencers can broaden your reach:

- **Partner with Influencers**: Collaborate with individuals who have a significant following to share information about NIK deficiency and advocate for awareness.
- **Challenge and Engage**: Create challenges that encourage users to participate in awareness activities, such as sharing facts or their own stories.

Conclusion

Education and awareness are essential in transforming the landscape for individuals living with NIK deficiency. By reducing stigma, encouraging early diagnosis, and empowering individuals, we can create a more informed and supportive community. Through local initiatives, media engagement, and social media campaigns, we can significantly enhance public understanding of this condition. In the next chapter, we will explore how NIK deficiency is managed across different countries, highlighting international perspectives and practices.

Chapter 15: International Perspectives

NIK deficiency, while a specific condition, affects individuals around the globe, highlighting the diverse ways in which different countries approach its management, treatment, and support. Understanding international perspectives on NIK deficiency can provide valuable insights into effective practices and highlight the disparities that exist in healthcare systems. This chapter will explore how NIK deficiency is managed in various countries, discuss differences in access to treatment, and share compelling stories from around the world.

How NIK Deficiency is Managed Globally
1. Variations in Diagnosis and Treatment Protocols

- **Diagnostic Practices**: In countries with advanced healthcare systems, such as the United States and many European nations, genetic testing for NIK deficiency is increasingly common. Early and accurate diagnosis allows for timely interventions. Conversely, in some developing countries, access to such tests may be limited, resulting in delayed or incorrect diagnoses.

- **Treatment Approaches**: Treatment protocols vary widely. In North America, immunoglobulin replacement therapy is the standard approach, alongside proactive management of infections. In contrast, other regions may rely more on empirical antibiotic therapy due to limited resources or lack of access to specialized care.

2. Healthcare System Differences

- **Access to Care**: Countries with universal healthcare systems often provide better access to specialized care for individuals with NIK deficiency. In the UK, for example, individuals have access to immunology specialists through the National Health Service (NHS), facilitating comprehensive management of their condition. In contrast, in the United States, the quality of care can vary significantly based on insurance coverage, potentially leaving some individuals without necessary treatments.

- **Insurance and Cost**: In some countries, the financial burden of treatments like immunoglobulin therapy can be overwhelming. In countries with robust healthcare policies, such costs may be covered, while in others, out-of-pocket expenses can lead to treatment gaps.

Stories from Around the World

1. The United States: A Multifaceted Approach

In the U.S., families dealing with NIK deficiency often find support through specialized clinics. One family, the Garcias, share their journey of navigating the complex healthcare landscape. With a child diagnosed at a young age, they learned to advocate for access to immunoglobulin therapy. Their experience highlights the importance of having a knowledgeable healthcare team and the emotional toll that comes with managing a chronic condition.

2. United Kingdom: Community Support Systems

In the UK, individuals with NIK deficiency often benefit from the National Health Service and various patient advocacy organizations. Sarah, a young adult with NIK deficiency, recounts her experience of joining a local support group. These community connections not only provided her with practical advice on managing her condition but also fostered friendships that made her journey feel less isolating.

3. India: Overcoming Barriers

In India, the story of Rahul illustrates the challenges faced by individuals with NIK deficiency in a resource-limited setting. Diagnosed late due to a lack of awareness among healthcare providers, Rahul's family fought to access appropriate care. Their persistence led them to an immunology clinic where they finally received proper treatment. Rahul's story emphasizes the need for increased education and awareness about immunodeficiencies in underserved areas.

Conclusion

The global landscape of NIK deficiency management reveals both the progress made and the challenges that persist. Understanding these international perspectives enriches our knowledge of effective practices and underscores the necessity for advocacy in regions where care is lacking. By learning from one another, we can work toward a more equitable approach to managing NIK deficiency worldwide.

In the next chapter, we will explore real-life case studies that provide deeper insights into the experiences of individuals with NIK deficiency, showcasing resilience and the diverse strategies employed to navigate daily challenges.

Chapter 16: Case Studies

Real-life experiences of individuals living with NIK deficiency can illuminate the challenges and triumphs associated with managing this condition. Through personal stories, we can better understand the emotional, social, and medical complexities that accompany NIK deficiency. This chapter presents several case studies that highlight different aspects of living with this condition, the lessons learned, and the resilience exhibited by those affected.

Case Study 1: Emily's Journey to Diagnosis

Background: Emily, a 10-year-old girl from a suburban town, began experiencing recurrent infections and extreme fatigue. Initially dismissed by her pediatrician as common childhood illnesses, her condition worsened over several months.

Diagnosis: After a particularly severe bout of pneumonia, her parents insisted on further testing. Blood work revealed low immunoglobulin levels, and genetic testing confirmed NIK deficiency. The diagnosis came as both a relief and a challenge, as her family now faced the task of understanding the condition and its implications.

Lessons Learned: Emily's story underscores the importance of advocacy in healthcare. Her parents learned to trust their instincts and push for answers when their daughter's health was at stake. They became proactive in seeking out specialists and joined a support group for families dealing with immunodeficiencies. This community provided them with valuable information and emotional support, significantly easing their journey.

Case Study 2: Raj's Support System

Background: Raj, a 28-year-old man from India, was diagnosed with NIK deficiency in his late teens after experiencing frequent hospitalizations for infections. With limited access to specialized care, Raj struggled to manage his condition and often felt isolated.

Community Engagement: Over the years, Raj sought out local support groups, eventually becoming a leader within them. He organized awareness campaigns in his community, focusing on educating both healthcare providers and the general public about NIK deficiency.

Impact: Raj's activism not only empowered him but also improved access to information and resources for others facing similar challenges. His journey illustrates the transformative power of community support and the importance of raising awareness in underrepresented areas.

Case Study 3: Maria's Holistic Approach

Background: Maria, a 35-year-old woman from Brazil, was diagnosed with NIK deficiency after a long history of autoimmune issues and chronic infections. Frustrated with traditional treatment options, she turned to holistic therapies to complement her medical regimen.

Integrative Practices: Maria incorporated yoga, meditation, and a nutrient-rich diet into her daily routine. She found that these practices helped reduce her stress levels and improve her overall well-being. Working closely with her healthcare providers, she combined these approaches with her prescribed treatments, leading to better health outcomes.

Takeaway: Maria's experience highlights the potential benefits of a holistic approach to managing chronic conditions. While medical treatment is essential, complementary therapies can play a significant role in enhancing quality of life and emotional resilience.

Case Study 4: Alex's Transition to Adult Care

Background: Alex, a 19-year-old college student in Canada, faced a significant transition as he moved from pediatric to adult healthcare services. Diagnosed with NIK deficiency at a young age, he was used to a familiar pediatric team that understood his history.

Navigating the System: The transition was daunting. Alex encountered challenges in establishing care with new providers who were less familiar with his condition. Recognizing the need for advocacy, he prepared a comprehensive health summary to share with his new healthcare team, ensuring continuity of care.

Outcome: By taking charge of his health and being proactive in his communication with new providers, Alex successfully navigated this transition. His story emphasizes the importance of preparation and advocacy when moving to adult healthcare systems.

Conclusion

These case studies illustrate the diverse experiences of individuals living with NIK deficiency. From the importance of early diagnosis and proactive advocacy to the value of community support and holistic approaches, each story offers unique insights into the multifaceted nature of this condition. By sharing these narratives, we foster a deeper understanding of the challenges faced by those with NIK deficiency and inspire resilience in the face of adversity.

In the next chapter, we will discuss strategies for preparing for the future, including planning for transitions in care, family planning, and long-term health monitoring.

Chapter 17: Preparing for the Future

Preparing for the future is crucial for individuals with NIK deficiency and their families. This chapter discusses the essential aspects of planning for transitions in care, family planning considerations, and the importance of long-term health monitoring. By being proactive and informed, patients can navigate the complexities of their condition more effectively and enhance their quality of life.

Planning for Transitions in Care

As individuals with NIK deficiency grow older, they will inevitably transition from pediatric to adult healthcare systems. This shift can be challenging, especially since adult care may not be as familiar with the nuances of NIK deficiency as pediatric specialists. Here are strategies to ensure a smooth transition:

1. **Start Early**: Begin the transition process around the age of 16 to 18. This timeframe allows for gradual exposure to adult healthcare settings while still having support from pediatric providers.

2. **Build a Comprehensive Health Summary**: Create a document summarizing medical history, treatments, and medications. This summary should include details about NIK deficiency, any coexisting conditions, and past treatments. This document will be invaluable when meeting new healthcare providers.

3. **Research Adult Specialists**: Identify adult healthcare providers who have experience with immunodeficiencies. Seek recommendations from pediatric specialists and patient advocacy groups.

4. **Prepare for Appointments**: Encourage the individual to take an active role in their healthcare by preparing questions and discussing concerns during appointments. This practice fosters independence and engagement.

5. **Encourage Communication**: Establish an open line of communication between the patient, their family, and the new healthcare team. This dialogue ensures continuity of care and allows the new team to understand the patient's unique needs.

Considering Fertility and Family Planning Options

For individuals with NIK deficiency, understanding the implications of their condition on fertility and family planning is essential. Here are some considerations:

1. **Consult Healthcare Providers**: Discuss reproductive health and family planning options with healthcare providers early on. This conversation can help address concerns about the impact of NIK deficiency on pregnancy and parenting.

2. **Genetic Counseling**: For those considering starting a family, genetic counseling can provide valuable insights into the inheritance patterns of NIK deficiency. Counselors can help assess risks and explore options for family planning.

3. **Health Monitoring During Pregnancy**: If planning a pregnancy, it is vital to collaborate with both an obstetrician and a specialist familiar with immunodeficiencies. Close monitoring during pregnancy can help manage health concerns that may arise.

4. **Support Networks**: Connecting with support groups for parents with immunodeficiencies can offer guidance and shared experiences, helping to navigate the challenges of parenting with a chronic condition.

Long-Term Health Monitoring

Regular health monitoring is crucial for individuals with NIK deficiency to manage their condition effectively. This section outlines key components of long-term health monitoring:

1. **Routine Check-Ups**: Establish a schedule for routine check-ups with healthcare providers to monitor immune function and assess any new symptoms. Regular visits can help catch potential complications early.

2. **Vaccination Awareness**: Stay informed about recommended vaccinations, as individuals with NIK deficiency may require specific immunizations to help prevent infections. Discuss vaccination plans with healthcare providers.

3. **Tracking Symptoms**: Maintain a symptom diary to track any recurrent infections, fatigue levels, or other changes in health. This documentation can assist healthcare providers in tailoring treatment plans.

4. **Lifestyle Adjustments**: Encourage ongoing attention to lifestyle factors that support immune health, including nutrition, exercise, and stress management. Regularly reassess these aspects to ensure they align with evolving health needs.

5. **Mental Health Support**: Recognize the importance of mental health monitoring. Encourage access to mental health resources to address anxiety or depression that may arise from living with a chronic condition.

Conclusion

Preparing for the future involves thoughtful planning and proactive management of NIK deficiency. By addressing transitions in care, considering family planning options, and committing to long-term health monitoring, individuals with NIK deficiency can navigate their health journey with confidence. Empowering patients and their families through education and support will help them embrace the future with resilience and hope.

In the next chapter, we will explore dietary considerations that play a crucial role in supporting immune health and overall well-being for individuals with NIK deficiency.

Chapter 18: Dietary Considerations

Nutrition plays a pivotal role in supporting the immune system, especially for individuals with NIK deficiency. A well-balanced diet can help manage symptoms, enhance immune function, and improve overall quality of life. This chapter will explore the importance of dietary choices, recommended nutritional supplements, and practical meal planning tips to empower individuals and families in their journey toward better health.

Importance of a Balanced Diet for Immune Health

A balanced diet provides the essential nutrients that the body needs to function optimally. For individuals with NIK deficiency, certain dietary considerations can make a significant difference in managing their condition:

1. **Macronutrients**: The body requires carbohydrates, proteins, and fats to sustain energy levels, repair tissues, and support immune function. A varied diet that includes whole grains, lean proteins, healthy fats, and plenty of fruits and vegetables is crucial.

2. **Micronutrients**: Vitamins and minerals play critical roles in immune health. Deficiencies in key nutrients can impair immune responses, making individuals more susceptible to infections. Focus on foods rich in:

- **Vitamin C**: Found in citrus fruits, bell peppers, and broccoli, this vitamin supports the immune system by promoting the production of white blood cells.

- **Vitamin D**: Important for immune modulation, vitamin D can be obtained through fatty fish, fortified foods, and sunlight exposure.

- **Zinc**: Present in meat, shellfish, legumes, and seeds, zinc is essential for immune cell development and function.

- **Selenium**: Found in nuts (especially Brazil nuts), seafood, and whole grains, selenium helps protect cells from damage and supports immune responses.

Hydration

Nutritional Supplements That May Support Immunity

While a balanced diet is the foundation of good health, some individuals with NIK deficiency may benefit from specific nutritional supplements. Before starting any supplements, it's important to consult with a healthcare provider to tailor choices to individual needs. Common supplements include:

1. **Multivitamins**: A daily multivitamin can help fill potential gaps in nutrient intake, particularly for those who may struggle to maintain a varied diet.
2. **Vitamin D**: Supplementation may be necessary for those with limited sun exposure or dietary intake. Optimal vitamin D levels are linked to enhanced immune function.
3. **Probiotics**: These beneficial bacteria can support gut health, which is increasingly recognized as vital for a strong immune system. Look for probiotic strains that have been studied for their immune-supporting properties.
4. **Omega-3 Fatty Acids**: Found in fish oil and flaxseed oil, omega-3s have anti-inflammatory effects and may enhance immune function.
5. **Herbal Supplements**: Some herbs, such as echinacea and elderberry, are believed to support immune health. However, it's essential to approach herbal supplements with caution and consult a healthcare provider.

Recipes and Meal Planning Tips

Incorporating immune-supportive foods into daily meals can be both enjoyable and beneficial. Here are some tips and easy recipes to promote healthy eating habits:

Meal Planning Tips

1. **Create a Weekly Menu**: Plan meals for the week, ensuring a variety of nutrients. Include fruits, vegetables, whole grains, lean proteins, and healthy fats in each meal.

2. **Batch Cooking**: Prepare larger portions of meals and freeze them for easy access during busy times. This approach helps maintain healthy eating without the stress of daily cooking.

3. **Snack Smart**: Choose snacks that provide nutritional value, such as fresh fruit, yogurt, nuts, or vegetable sticks with hummus.

4. **Mindful Eating**: Encourage individuals to practice mindful eating by focusing on the meal, savoring each bite, and recognizing hunger and fullness cues.

Sample Recipes

Immune-Boosting Smoothie

- Ingredients: 1 banana, 1 cup spinach, 1/2 cup Greek yogurt, 1/2 cup orange juice, and 1 tablespoon chia seeds.
- Instructions: Blend all ingredients until smooth. This smoothie is rich in vitamins, protein, and healthy fats.

Quinoa Salad with Roasted Vegetables

- Ingredients: 1 cup cooked quinoa, 1 cup assorted roasted vegetables (bell peppers, zucchini, carrots), 1/4 cup chickpeas, and a dressing of olive oil, lemon juice, salt, and pepper.
- Instructions: Mix all ingredients in a bowl and serve chilled or at room temperature. This dish is high in protein and fiber.

Baked Salmon with Sweet Potatoes

- Ingredients: 1 salmon fillet, 1 medium sweet potato, olive oil, garlic, and herbs (like rosemary or thyme).
- Instructions: Preheat the oven to 400°F (200°C). Coat the salmon with olive oil, garlic, and herbs. Bake alongside cubed sweet potatoes for 20-25 minutes. Rich in omega-3s and vitamins A and C.

Conclusion

Dietary considerations are essential for individuals with NIK deficiency, as proper nutrition supports immune health and overall well-being. By focusing on a balanced diet, incorporating nutritional supplements when necessary, and engaging in mindful meal planning, individuals can take proactive steps toward managing their condition.

In the next chapter, we will explore holistic approaches to health and well-being, including complementary therapies and mind-body practices that can enhance the quality of life for those living with NIK deficiency.

Chapter 19: Holistic Approaches

In the journey of managing NIK deficiency, holistic approaches can play a vital role in enhancing well-being and improving quality of life. These methods focus not only on the physical aspects of health but also on emotional, mental, and spiritual dimensions. This chapter will explore complementary therapies, mind-body practices, and the importance of caution and consultation with healthcare providers.

Complementary Therapies and Their Role

Complementary therapies can be used alongside traditional medical treatments to support overall health. These therapies can help alleviate symptoms, reduce stress, and promote a sense of control and well-being. Some notable complementary therapies include:

1. **Acupuncture**: This ancient Chinese practice involves inserting thin needles into specific points on the body. Acupuncture may help reduce pain and improve immune function by promoting balance in the body's energy pathways.

2. **Massage Therapy**: Therapeutic massage can relieve tension, reduce anxiety, and improve circulation. Regular massage sessions can provide relaxation and stress relief, which are particularly beneficial for those dealing with chronic health conditions.

3. **Herbal Medicine**: Certain herbs, such as echinacea, astragalus, and ginger, may offer immune-boosting properties. However, it's crucial to consult with a healthcare provider before incorporating herbal remedies, as they can interact with conventional medications.

4. **Aromatherapy**: Utilizing essential oils for therapeutic benefits can promote relaxation and emotional balance. Oils like lavender and chamomile are known for their calming effects, which can be beneficial in managing anxiety and stress.

5. **Physical Therapy**: Tailored physical therapy can improve strength, mobility, and overall physical function. It can be particularly beneficial for individuals experiencing fatigue or muscle weakness due to NIK deficiency.

Mind-Body Practices

Mind-body practices focus on the connection between mental and physical health. These practices can be particularly effective in reducing stress, enhancing emotional well-being, and promoting resilience. Some recommended mind-body practices include:

1. **Yoga**: This ancient practice combines physical postures, breathing techniques, and meditation. Yoga can improve flexibility, strength, and mental clarity while reducing stress and anxiety. Many individuals with chronic health conditions find that regular yoga practice enhances their overall sense of well-being.

2. **Meditation**: Mindfulness meditation encourages individuals to focus on the present moment and cultivate awareness without judgment. Regular meditation practice can reduce stress, enhance emotional regulation, and improve overall mental health.

3. **Tai Chi**: Often described as "meditation in motion," Tai Chi involves slow, deliberate movements and deep breathing. This practice can improve balance, reduce stress, and promote relaxation.

4. **Breathing Exercises**: Simple breathing techniques can help manage stress and anxiety. Practices such as diaphragmatic breathing or the 4-7-8 technique can promote relaxation and improve mental clarity.

5. **Journaling**: Writing about thoughts and feelings can be a powerful tool for self-reflection and emotional processing. Journaling can help individuals identify stressors and develop coping strategies, ultimately leading to improved emotional well-being.

Caution and Consultation with Healthcare Providers

While holistic approaches can be beneficial, it is essential to approach them with caution. Here are some key considerations:

1. **Consultation is Key**: Always discuss any complementary therapies or mind-body practices with your healthcare provider. This ensures that they are safe and appropriate for your specific condition and treatment plan.

2. **Individual Responses Vary**: Everyone responds differently to holistic approaches. What works for one individual may not work for another. It's important to find what resonates with you and supports your health journey.

3. **Avoid Replacement of Conventional Treatments**: Complementary therapies should not replace conventional medical treatments but rather serve as an adjunct to enhance overall well-being. Ensure that any holistic approach you consider complements your existing treatment plan.

4. **Quality and Safety**: When exploring supplements or herbal remedies, choose high-quality products from reputable sources. Some herbal products can interact with medications, so it's crucial to verify their safety with a healthcare professional.

5. **Listen to Your Body**: Pay attention to how your body responds to any new practice or treatment. If something doesn't feel right, discontinue the practice and consult your healthcare provider.

Conclusion

Holistic approaches can provide valuable support in managing NIK deficiency, addressing not only physical symptoms but also emotional and mental well-being. By exploring complementary therapies and engaging in mind-body practices, individuals can enhance their quality of life and promote resilience.

In the next chapter, we will delve into understanding research publications, empowering you to interpret scientific studies on NIK deficiency and stay informed about new findings. This knowledge will help you make informed decisions about your health and well-being.

Chapter 20: Understanding Research Publications

In the ever-evolving landscape of medical science, staying informed about research related to NIK deficiency is crucial. This chapter will guide you on how to interpret scientific studies, understand their relevance, and find resources for ongoing education. By becoming adept at evaluating research publications, you can empower yourself to make informed decisions regarding your health and treatment options.

How to Interpret Scientific Studies on NIK Deficiency

Understanding scientific research can seem daunting, but breaking it down into manageable components can clarify the information. Here are key aspects to consider when reading research publications:

1. **Abstract**: The abstract summarizes the study's objectives, methods, results, and conclusions. It provides a quick overview of what the study is about and its significance.

2. **Introduction**: This section outlines the background of the research, including previous studies and the rationale behind the current investigation. It sets the stage for understanding why the study was conducted.

3. **Methods**: The methods section details how the study was conducted, including the design, participants, and data collection techniques. Pay attention to the sample size and whether the study was randomized, as these factors impact the reliability of the results.

4. **Results**: Here, the authors present the findings of the study, often accompanied by charts, graphs, or tables. Focus on the key results that are directly related to NIK deficiency, noting any statistical significance.

5. **Discussion**: In the discussion section, researchers interpret the results, explaining their implications and how they relate to existing knowledge. This is also where limitations of the study are discussed, providing context for the findings.

6. **Conclusion**: The conclusion summarizes the main findings and suggests future research directions. It may also offer practical implications for individuals affected by NIK deficiency.

7. **References**: Check the reference list for the studies cited. This can help you identify additional resources and context related to the research topic.

Importance of Staying Informed About New Findings

Staying updated on research is vital for several reasons:

1. **Advancements in Treatment**: Research findings can lead to new therapies and management strategies for NIK deficiency. Understanding these advancements can help you discuss options with your healthcare provider.

2. **Personalized Care**: As research progresses, personalized medicine becomes increasingly relevant. Knowing the latest studies can help you advocate for treatments tailored to your specific needs.

3. **Empowerment**: Being informed allows you to take an active role in your health management. It enhances your ability to make informed decisions and engage in meaningful discussions with healthcare providers.

4. **Community and Support**: Sharing knowledge about recent research with support groups or communities can foster a sense of empowerment among individuals with NIK deficiency. It helps create a well-informed network that can advocate for better care and awareness.

Resources for Ongoing Education

Here are some valuable resources for accessing research publications and staying informed:

1. **PubMed**: A free database of scientific studies in the biomedical field. You can search for articles specifically related to NIK deficiency, immunology, and more.

2. **Google Scholar**: An accessible search engine for scholarly literature across various disciplines. It's a great tool for finding articles, theses, and books.

3. **Professional Journals**: Journals like the *Journal of Allergy and Clinical Immunology* and *Clinical Immunology* publish research on immunodeficiencies. Subscribing to these journals or checking their websites can keep you updated.

4. **Patient Advocacy Organizations**: Many organizations focused on immunodeficiencies and rare diseases provide educational resources, newsletters, and updates on research findings.

5. **Conferences and Webinars**: Attending conferences related to immunology can provide insights into cutting-edge research. Many organizations offer webinars that discuss the latest findings and treatment approaches.

6. **Social Media and Online Communities**: Platforms like Twitter and Facebook often feature discussions and updates from researchers and healthcare professionals. Joining groups dedicated to NIK deficiency or immunology can help you connect with others and share knowledge.

Conclusion

Understanding research publications is an empowering tool in managing NIK deficiency. By learning how to interpret scientific studies and staying informed about the latest findings, you can advocate for your health and engage more effectively with your healthcare team. In the next chapter, we will explore legal rights and resources available to patients, ensuring that you are well-informed about your rights and the support systems in place.

Chapter 21: Legal Rights and Resources

Navigating the complexities of living with NIK deficiency involves not only understanding the medical and psychological aspects of the condition but also recognizing your legal rights and available resources. This chapter aims to empower you with knowledge about patient rights, discrimination laws, legal assistance, and advocacy organizations that can support you in your journey.

Patient Rights Regarding Treatment and Discrimination

As a patient with NIK deficiency, it's essential to know your rights. These rights vary by country and region but generally include the following:

1. **Right to Informed Consent**: You have the right to receive comprehensive information about your diagnosis, treatment options, potential risks, and benefits. This information should be provided in a manner that you can understand, enabling you to make informed decisions about your care.

2. **Right to Non-Discrimination**: Under various laws, including the Americans with Disabilities Act (ADA) in the United States, individuals with chronic health conditions, including immunodeficiencies, are protected from discrimination in employment, public services, and accommodations. This means you should not face unjust treatment due to your condition.

3. **Right to Privacy**: You have the right to confidentiality regarding your medical records and personal health information. Healthcare providers must ensure that your information is kept secure and shared only with your consent.

4. **Right to Access Care**: You are entitled to receive necessary medical care without unreasonable delays. This includes having access to specialists and treatments relevant to your NIK deficiency.

5. **Right to Appeal**: If you encounter denial of services, treatments, or insurance claims, you have the right to appeal those decisions. Familiarize yourself with the process to advocate for your needs effectively.

Resources for Legal Assistance

Understanding your rights is one step; knowing where to turn for help is another. Here are resources to assist you in navigating legal matters related to NIK deficiency:

1. **Legal Aid Organizations**: Many communities have legal aid services that offer free or low-cost legal assistance to individuals facing discrimination or issues related to healthcare access. Search for local legal aid organizations that focus on healthcare or disability rights.

2. **Disability Rights Organizations**: Groups such as the National Disability Rights Network (NDRN) in the United States provide information, advocacy, and legal assistance for individuals with disabilities. They can help you understand your rights and the resources available to you.

3. **Patient Advocacy Groups**: Many organizations focus on specific conditions or immunodeficiencies. These groups often have resources and support networks to assist with navigating healthcare and legal issues. They can also guide you on how to address discrimination.

4. **Ombudsman Services**: Some regions have ombudsman services that mediate disputes between patients and healthcare providers. They can offer guidance on how to resolve complaints or disputes related to care.

Advocacy Organizations and How to Get Involved

Engaging with advocacy organizations can provide additional support, information, and resources. Here's how you can get involved:

1. **Join Local or National Organizations**: Many organizations focus on immunodeficiencies or general health advocacy. Joining these groups can connect you with resources, community events, and networks of individuals facing similar challenges.

2. **Participate in Awareness Campaigns**: Many advocacy groups run awareness campaigns to educate the public and policymakers about conditions like NIK deficiency. Participating in these campaigns can amplify your voice and help raise awareness.

3. **Volunteer for Advocacy Efforts**: If you're passionate about patient rights, consider volunteering with an advocacy organization. Your experiences and insights can contribute to efforts aimed at improving healthcare access and quality for individuals with NIK deficiency.

4. **Engage in Policy Advocacy**: Many organizations focus on influencing healthcare policy. Engaging in advocacy at local, state, or national levels can help shape legislation that impacts individuals with immunodeficiencies.

Conclusion

Understanding your legal rights and available resources is essential for navigating the challenges of living with NIK deficiency. By knowing your rights, seeking legal assistance when necessary, and engaging with advocacy organizations, you can empower yourself and others in the community. In the next chapter, we will explore future directions in treatment, examining potential breakthroughs and the evolving landscape of personalized medicine in the management of NIK deficiency.

Chapter 22: Future Directions in Treatment

As our understanding of NIK deficiency continues to evolve, so too does the landscape of potential treatments. This chapter will explore promising breakthroughs in immunology, the emerging role of personalized medicine, and the future challenges and hopes for managing NIK deficiency.

Potential Breakthroughs in Immunology

Recent advancements in immunology offer exciting possibilities for treating NIK deficiency. Research in this field has focused on several key areas:

1. **Gene Therapy**: One of the most groundbreaking approaches being investigated is gene therapy, which aims to correct or replace the faulty genes responsible for NIK deficiency. While still in experimental stages, preliminary studies have shown that gene therapy could potentially restore normal immune function in affected individuals, offering a long-term solution rather than ongoing treatments.

2. **Biologics**: The development of biologic therapies—medications derived from living organisms—has gained traction in the treatment of various immunodeficiencies. These treatments can specifically target pathways in the immune response that are disrupted by NIK deficiency, providing more effective management of symptoms and reducing the frequency of infections.

3. **Immunomodulators**: These drugs help adjust or modulate the immune system's activity. Research is ongoing into how specific immunomodulators could help enhance immune function in individuals with NIK deficiency, potentially decreasing susceptibility to infections and improving overall health.

Role of Personalized Medicine

Personalized medicine, which tailors treatment plans to the individual characteristics of each patient, is increasingly becoming a cornerstone in the management of many health conditions, including NIK deficiency. This approach includes:

1. **Genetic Profiling**: By analyzing the genetic makeup of patients, healthcare providers can better understand how NIK deficiency manifests in different individuals. This knowledge allows for customized treatment plans that consider specific genetic variations and responses to medications.

2. **Tailored Therapies**: As our understanding of individual variations in immune responses grows, therapies can be fine-tuned to maximize effectiveness and minimize side effects. Personalized approaches may include selecting the most suitable immunoglobulin therapies or optimizing dosage regimens based on genetic markers.

3. **Patient-Centered Care**: Personalized medicine emphasizes collaboration between patients and healthcare providers. Patients become active participants in their treatment decisions, leading to more effective management strategies and improved adherence to therapies.

Future Challenges and Hopes

While advancements in treatment offer great promise, several challenges remain:

1. **Access to New Therapies**: As innovative treatments emerge, ensuring equitable access to these therapies will be critical. This includes addressing disparities in healthcare systems and making sure that all patients can benefit from the latest advancements.

2. **Research Funding and Support**: Continued investment in research is essential for uncovering new treatments and understanding the complexities of NIK deficiency. Advocacy for funding and support for research initiatives will be crucial in driving future breakthroughs.

3. **Patient Education**: As new treatments and approaches are developed, educating patients and healthcare providers about these innovations will be vital. Empowering individuals with knowledge about their options can lead to better health outcomes and enhanced quality of life.

4. **Long-Term Monitoring**: As treatment strategies evolve, ongoing monitoring will be essential to assess their effectiveness and identify any long-term implications. Regular follow-ups and assessments will help ensure that patients receive the best possible care.

Conclusion

The future of treating NIK deficiency is bright, with promising breakthroughs in immunology and a growing emphasis on personalized medicine. While challenges remain, the continued dedication of researchers, healthcare providers, and advocates will pave the way for more effective management strategies. In the following chapter, we will explore how to collaborate with healthcare providers to build a strong relationship and create effective care plans, ensuring the best possible outcomes for individuals living with NIK deficiency.

Chapter 23: Collaborating with Healthcare Providers

Building a strong, effective relationship with healthcare providers is essential for managing NIK deficiency. This collaboration ensures that patients receive comprehensive, personalized care tailored to their specific needs. In this chapter, we will discuss the importance of communication and trust in the patient-provider relationship, as well as how to create an effective care plan.

Building a Strong Relationship with Your Medical Team

Choosing the Right Healthcare Providers

Finding knowledgeable and experienced healthcare providers who understand NIK deficiency is crucial. Look for specialists in immunology or genetics who are familiar with the latest research and treatment options. A supportive primary care physician can also play a key role in coordinating care.

Establishing Open Lines of Communication

Effective communication is the cornerstone of a successful healthcare partnership. Be open about your symptoms, concerns, and treatment goals. Regularly updating your providers on any changes in your health can help them make informed decisions.

Setting Expectations

Discuss your expectations for care, including desired outcomes, preferred treatment options, and any personal preferences. This conversation can help ensure that everyone is on the same page regarding your health journey.

Importance of Communication and Trust

Building Trust

Trust is fundamental in any healthcare relationship. Patients should feel comfortable discussing sensitive topics, asking questions, and expressing concerns. A good provider will listen empathetically and validate your experiences.

Being an Active Participant

Engage actively in your care. This means asking questions, seeking clarification on treatment plans, and advocating for your needs. When patients take an active role, it fosters a sense of empowerment and control over their health.

Documenting Your Health Journey

Keep a detailed record of your symptoms, treatments, and any side effects you experience. This information can help healthcare providers understand your condition better and adjust treatments as necessary.

Creating an Effective Care Plan

Personalized Care Plans

Work with your healthcare team to develop a personalized care plan that addresses your unique needs. This plan should outline treatment goals, medication schedules, lifestyle modifications, and any necessary follow-up appointments.

Regular Reviews and Adjustments

Your care plan should be a living document, reviewed and updated regularly. As your condition changes or new treatments become available, adjustments may be needed to optimize your management strategy.

Incorporating Multidisciplinary Care

Consider a multidisciplinary approach involving various specialists, such as immunologists, nutritionists, and mental health professionals. This collaborative approach ensures comprehensive care that addresses all aspects of living with NIK deficiency.

Emergency Preparedness

Include emergency plans in your care plan, detailing what to do in case of infections or other acute issues related to NIK deficiency. Make sure your family and caregivers are aware of these plans.

Building a Support Network

Involving Family and Friends

Educate your loved ones about NIK deficiency so they can better understand your experiences and provide support. Encourage them to accompany you to appointments when possible, as having an advocate can be incredibly beneficial.

Utilizing Support Groups

Connect with support groups for individuals with NIK deficiency or similar conditions. These communities can offer emotional support, practical advice, and shared experiences that can enhance your journey.

Advocacy and Involvement

Engage in advocacy efforts to raise awareness about NIK deficiency. By collaborating with healthcare providers and organizations, you can contribute to research and improvements in treatment options for yourself and others.

Conclusion

Collaboration with healthcare providers is essential for effective management of NIK deficiency. By building strong relationships based on communication and trust, and by actively participating in your care, you can create a personalized care plan that addresses your unique needs. In the next chapter, we will explore how community involvement can enhance your support network and promote advocacy for those affected by NIK deficiency.

Chapter 24: Community Involvement

Community involvement is a powerful tool for individuals living with NIK deficiency and their families. Engaging with your community not only enhances your support network but also helps raise awareness, improve access to resources, and foster a culture of understanding and advocacy. This chapter explores various ways to get involved, including volunteering, participating in local health initiatives, and building a supportive community network.

Volunteering and Advocacy Opportunities

Finding Volunteer Opportunities

Many organizations focused on immune deficiencies and chronic health conditions offer volunteer opportunities. This could range from administrative support to event organization. Participating in these activities can provide valuable experience and connect you with others who share similar experiences.

Advocating for Awareness

Advocacy plays a critical role in raising awareness about NIK deficiency. Engage in campaigns that educate the public, healthcare providers, and policymakers about the challenges faced by individuals with NIK deficiency. This could involve writing articles, participating in local health fairs, or speaking at community events.

Participating in Fundraising

Fundraising initiatives are essential for supporting research and resources for individuals with NIK deficiency. Consider organizing or participating in events such as walks, runs, or benefit concerts. These events not only raise funds but also promote community engagement and awareness.

Engaging with Local Health Initiatives

Collaborating with Local Healthcare Providers

Work with local clinics and hospitals to organize health seminars or informational sessions on NIK deficiency. These initiatives can help educate healthcare professionals and the community, fostering a more informed environment for those affected.

Joining Health Initiatives

Many communities have health initiatives focused on wellness, preventive care, and chronic illness management. Joining these initiatives can provide access to resources, workshops, and support groups tailored to the needs of individuals with NIK deficiency.

Participating in Health Screenings

Engage in or promote health screenings organized by local health organizations. Early detection and intervention are vital for managing NIK deficiency effectively. These screenings can help raise awareness and encourage community members to seek medical attention when needed.

Building a Supportive Community Network

Creating Support Groups

Establish local support groups for individuals and families affected by NIK deficiency. These groups provide a safe space to share experiences, resources, and coping strategies. They can also foster friendships and support among those facing similar challenges.

Utilizing Online Communities

In addition to local groups, online communities can be invaluable for connecting with others around the globe. Social media platforms and dedicated forums can provide ongoing support, resources, and information on the latest research and developments related to NIK deficiency.

Organizing Community Events

Host or participate in community events that raise awareness about NIK deficiency. Consider informational workshops, health fairs, or family days focused on health education. These events can engage the community while promoting understanding and support for individuals affected by NIK deficiency.

Fostering Inclusivity and Awareness

Educational Campaigns

Launch educational campaigns that inform the community about NIK deficiency, its symptoms, and the importance of early diagnosis. Distributing brochures, creating informational websites, and utilizing social media can effectively spread awareness.

Encouraging Inclusivity

Work to foster an inclusive environment in schools, workplaces, and community organizations. Encourage discussions about health issues, including NIK deficiency, to promote understanding and support for those affected.

Partnering with Local Organizations

Collaborate with organizations that focus on chronic illnesses, disabilities, and health education. These partnerships can amplify your efforts, bringing more visibility to NIK deficiency and helping to create a more supportive community environment.

Conclusion

Community involvement is essential for fostering support, raising awareness, and improving the lives of individuals affected by NIK deficiency. By volunteering, engaging with local health initiatives, and building a supportive network, you can make a significant impact not only in your life but also in the lives of others facing similar challenges. In the final chapter, we will reflect on the key insights from this book and offer an inspirational message for those affected by NIK deficiency, encouraging continued awareness and support.

Chapter 25: Conclusion and Hope

As we conclude this journey through the intricacies of NIK deficiency, it is essential to reflect on the knowledge gained and the path forward. This book aimed to provide a comprehensive understanding of NIK deficiency, highlighting its impact on individuals and families, while fostering a sense of community and hope.

Recap of Key Insights

1. **Understanding NIK Deficiency**: We have explored the definition, genetic basis, and prevalence of NIK deficiency. Understanding its roots allows for better diagnosis, management, and treatment.

2. **The Immune System's Role**: A deep dive into the immune system illuminated how NIK deficiency disrupts normal immune function, leading to increased susceptibility to infections and other complications.

3. **Holistic Management Strategies**: From individualized care plans to lifestyle adjustments, we have discussed various strategies to manage NIK deficiency effectively. Emphasizing nutrition, hygiene, and mental health are vital components of a comprehensive care approach.

4. **Advocacy and Awareness**: The importance of raising awareness about NIK deficiency cannot be overstated. Community involvement and education can significantly improve understanding and resources available for those affected.

5. **Research and Future Directions**: Ongoing research holds promise for new treatments and management strategies, from advancements in gene therapy to personalized medicine. Staying informed about these developments is crucial for hope and empowerment.

6. **Legal Rights and Resources**: Understanding patient rights and available resources is essential for navigating healthcare systems and ensuring access to appropriate care and support.

Inspirational Message for Those Affected

To everyone living with NIK deficiency, remember that you are not alone. Your journey may be challenging, but your resilience, strength, and determination are powerful. Embrace your story and share it with others; your experiences can inspire hope and understanding in those who may feel isolated.

For caregivers and family members, your support is invaluable. Together, you can create a nurturing environment that promotes health, wellness, and happiness. Your role is critical in advocating for better resources and understanding within your community.

Call to Action for Awareness and Research Support

As we close this chapter, I encourage you to take action. Engage with local and online communities, advocate for awareness, and support research initiatives aimed at improving the lives of those affected by NIK deficiency.

- **Volunteer**: Join organizations dedicated to immunodeficiencies, participate in fundraising events, or start local awareness campaigns.
- **Educate**: Share the information and insights gained from this book with friends, family, and your community. Awareness can drive change and create supportive environments.
- **Support Research**: Contribute to research organizations, participate in clinical trials if eligible, and stay informed about the latest developments in NIK deficiency and related fields.

Closing Thoughts

In the face of adversity, hope is a guiding light. Together, we can foster a world where those affected by NIK deficiency are understood, supported, and empowered to lead fulfilling lives. Thank you for embarking on this journey toward mastering NIK deficiency, and may we continue to strive for awareness, research, and community support for all who are impacted.